Sawsan Daoud
Mariem Damak
Chokri Mhiri

The parietal lobe: descriptive, functional and clinical anatomy

Sawsan Daoud
Mariem Damak
Chokri Mhiri

The parietal lobe: descriptive, functional and clinical anatomy

ScienciaScripts

Imprint

Cover image: www.ingimage.com

This book is a translation from the original published under ISBN 978-620-6-70399-0.

Publisher:
Sciencia Scripts
is a trademark of
Dodo Books Indian Ocean Ltd. and OmniScriptum S.R.L publishing group

120 High Road, East Finchley, London, N2 9ED, United Kingdom
Str. Armeneasca 28/1, office 1, Chisinau MD-2012, Republic of Moldova, Europe
Printed at: see last page
ISBN: 978-620-7-20729-9

The parietal lobe

Descriptive, functional and clinical anatomy

Table of contents

Introduction:

The parietal lobe is a highly developed structure in humans. It functions in close relation to other brain structures, as it is the seat of reception and integration of sensory and sensory information. This lobe thus constitutes a veritable crossroads between motor representations and sensory and sensory projections. This explains the richness of clinical symptomatology following damage to the parietal lobe. Indeed, although the sensory role of the parietal cortex is in the foreground, its functions are far more complex. To understand parietal symptomatology, we need to bear in mind that the parietal lobe is divided into three functional regions:

- The primary somato-sensitive area, whose lesion will cause contralateral elementary sensory disorders
- Secondary somato-sensory areas, which are responsible for deficits in the complex integration of sensory perceptions
- The tertiary areas of multi-modal sensory integration, whose lesion will result in complex deficits in several perceptual-cognitive modalities, as well as disorders of symbolic functions, depending on the location and laterality of the lesion. The right cerebral hemisphere controls thought and spatial memory, while the left hemisphere is concerned with episodic memory and symbolic thought.

Given the complexity of parietal symptomatology, we've taken an interest in this subject. We will study the anatomy and functional anatomy of the parietal lobe. We will also determine the various components of the parietal syndrome, while specifying the anatomo-clinical correlations.

The objectives of this work are:

1- Describe the anatomy and functional anatomy of the parietal lobe

2- Determining the various symptoms of parietal syndrome

3- Establishing anatomo-clinical correlations

4- Plan a diagnostic approach to symptoms suggestive of a parietal syndrome

1. Anatomy of the parietal lobe :

The parietal lobe is located in the upper and middle part of the cerebral hemisphere (Figure 1).

- On the outer side of the brain, this lobe is delimited :
  - Forward through the central or Rolando scissure
  - Backwards through the parieto-occipital sulcus and an imaginary line that continues this sulcus
  - Below, by the lateral scissure or scissure of sylvius and an imaginary line that continues this scissure to the occipital lobe

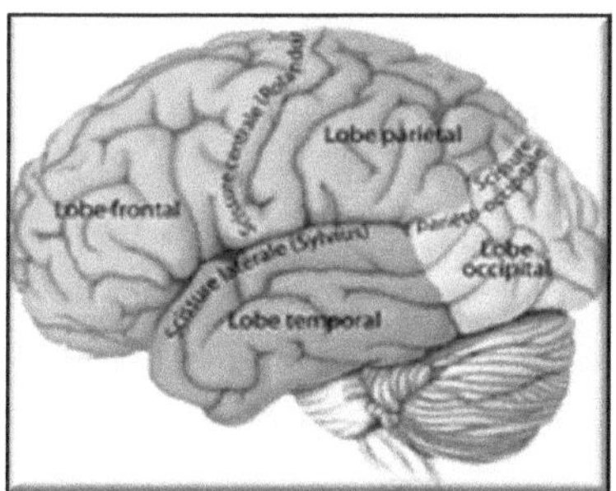

Figure 1Anatomical relationships of the parietal lobe

The T-shaped intraparietal sulcus divides the parietal lobe into 3 convolutions or gyri (Figure 2) (1) :

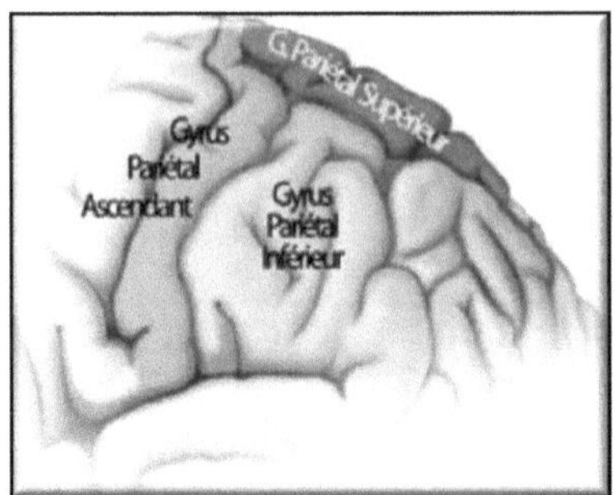

Figure 2Architecture of the parietal lobe

- <u>The ascending parietal convolution or post-central convolution:</u> located in the anterior part of the parietal lobe. It is bounded anteriorly by Rolando's scissure and posteriorly by the vertical branch of the intraparietal sulcus. It is formed by Brodmann's areas 3, 1, 2 (Figure 3). At its base, this gyrus has the parietal operculum above the lateral sulcus.

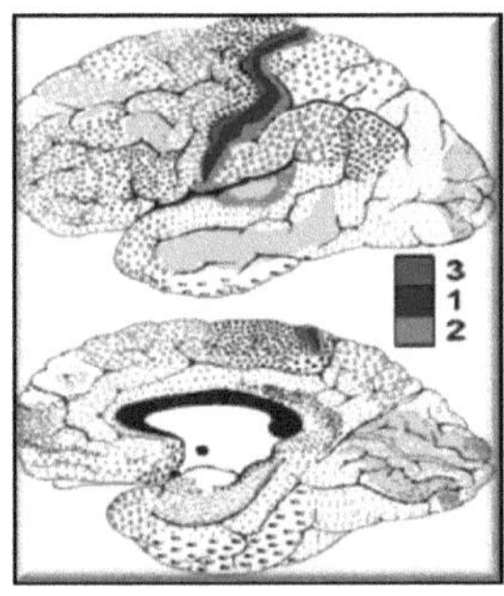

Figure 3The ascending parietal convolution

  - <u>The upper parietal convolution</u> (areas 5 and 7) is bounded at the bottom by the horizontal branch of the intraparietal sulcus (Figure 4). Internally, it forms the quadrilateral lobule or precuneus.

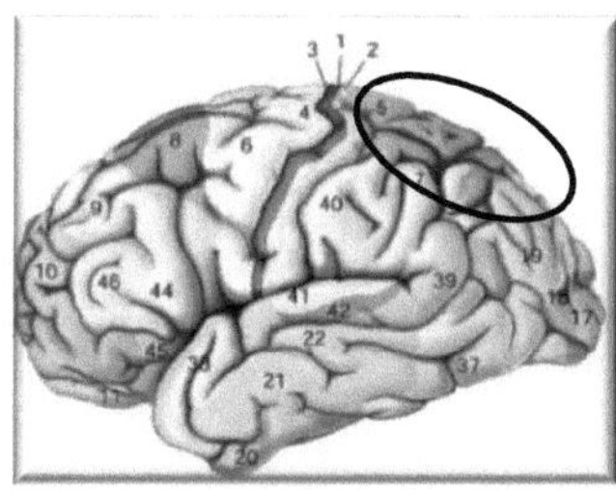

Figure 4The superior parietal convolution

- The inferior parietal convolution: split in two by Jensen's sulcus, which arises from the intraparietal sulcus: its anterior part forms the supra-marginal gyrus (Brodmann's area (AB) 40), which covers the upper end of the lateral sulcus, and its posterior part, the angular gyrus or curved fold (AB 39), which covers the inferior temporal sulcus (Figure 5).

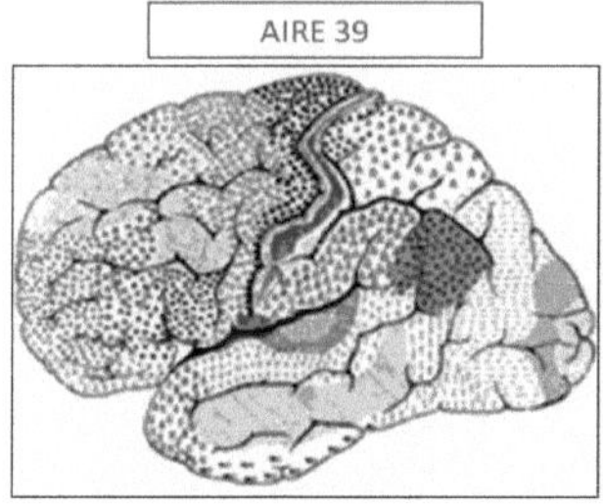

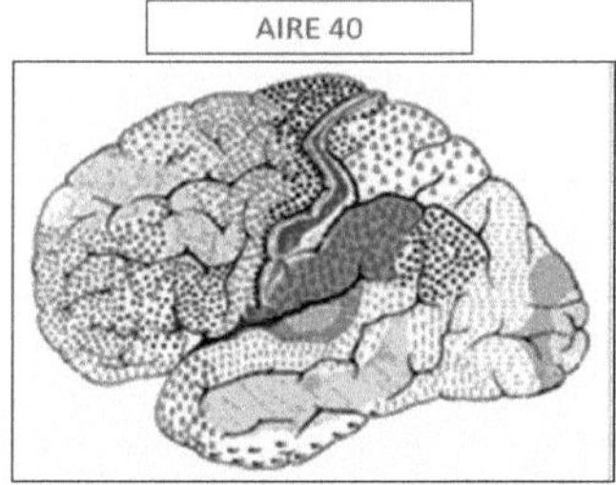

Figure 5The lower parietal convolution: AB 39 and AB 40

- On the inner surface of the hemisphere, the anterior limit of the parietal lobe is formed by an imaginary extension of Rolando's scissure, while the posterior limit is represented by the parieto-occipital sulcus. The inner surface of the parietal lobe includes the posterior part of the para-central lobule, formed by the medial part of the post-central gyrus, and behind it, the precuneus.

- Vascularization of the parietal lobe :

Vascularization of the parietal lobe depends on the anterior cerebral artery and the middle cerebral artery.

- Medial side: the paracentral and quadrilateral lobules are vascularized by the anterior cerebral artery.
- External face of the parietal lobe: vascularized by the middle cerebral artery

2. Functional anatomy of the parietal lobe :

Architecturally and functionally, the parietal lobe is divided into three functional regions:

2.1 Primary sensory area or somato-sensory cortex:

Formed by the ascending parietal convolution (AB 3,1 and 2). It receives afferents from the third neuron of the sensory pathway, originating from the posterolateral ventral nucleus of the thalamus. The representation of the various segments of the contralateral hemisphere is that of Penfield's homonculus. This is the sensory homonculus, with an inverted projection of the body, visible in the organization of the cortex. Indeed, the legs and trunk are represented in the midline, the arms and hands towards the middle of the gyrus, while the face is represented in the lower part of the postcentral gyrus (Figure 6) (2).

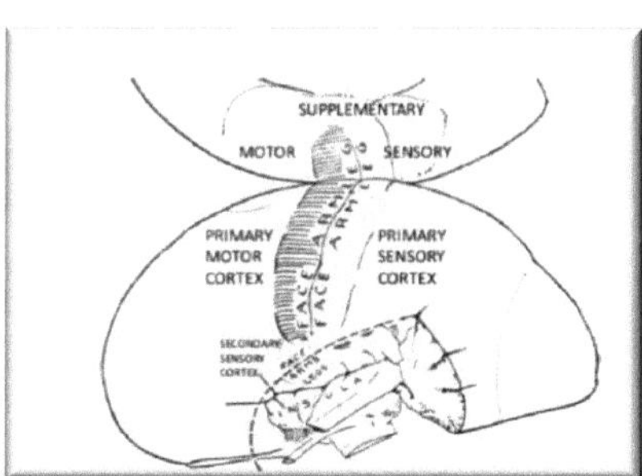

Figure 6The sensory homonculus

2.1.1 Brodmann area 3:

It is divided into area 3a and area 3b (3). Area 3a receives information from neuromuscular spindles. Area 3b receives information from cutaneous receptors. This area is highly granular and is considered to be the true primary somato-sensory cortex.

2.1.2 Brodmann area 1:

This area represents a peripheral receptive field confined to a finger. It responds only to stimuli applied to the skin of a finger.

2.1.3 Brodmann area 2:

Area 2 functional units have a multi-digital receptive field, and receive stimuli not only from the skin, but also from muscles and joint capsules. (2).

Each of AB 3, 1 and 2 contains neurons that project their axons into secondary somato-sensory areas.

2.2 Secondary somato-sensory areas :

Formed by the superior parietal convolution (AB 5 and 7) (2).

2.2.1 Brodmann's Area 5:

Brodmann's area 5 is located in the upper part of the parietal lobe, immediately posterior to the primary sensory cortex. It is involved in processing somato-sensory information, thus representing an association cortex. This area is activated during movements made by the contralateral upper limb under visual control.

2.2.2 *Brodmann area 7:*

This area also corresponds to an associative somato-sensory cortex. Located at the conjunction of perceptual (forward) and visual (backward) areas, it plays a role in visuo-perceptual coordination, integrating proprioceptive and visual information. It thus enables us to determine the relative position of an object in space in relation to the body or parts of it. It is also involved in prehension tasks (visually pursuing an object to grasp it).

2.3 Tertiary sensory integration areas :

Formed by the inferior parietal convolution (AB 39 and 40). These are multimodal integration areas: somato-sensory, vestibular, visual and symbolic. (4).

2.3.1 *Area 39: the angular gyrus or curved fold:*

Brodmann's area 39 corresponds to a junction between the occipital, parietal and temporal cortices. It surrounds the caudal end of the temporal sulcus. This area is bounded dorsally by the intra-parietal sulcus and rostrally by the supramarginal area (area 40). Its upper and posterior limit is bordered by the peristriatal cortex (area 19) and its lower limit by the occipitotemporal area (area 37). This area is anatomically distinct from one hemisphere to the other. The curved fold of the dominant parietal lobe plays an important role in language comprehension and reading.

2.3.2 *Area 40: supra-marginal gyrus:*

Brodmann's area 40 forms a junction between the parietal and temporal lobes. It is bounded by the intra-parietal sulcus, the inferior post-central sulcus and the lateral sulcus. It is also bordered by the angular gyrus below (area 39), the primary somato-sensory cortex above (area 2) and, at depth, by the subcentral area (43). This area is involved in knowledge of the existence of body parts and their spatial relationships.

3. Hemispheric asymmetries :

Neuropsychological data suggest a sequential analytical function for the left hemisphere and a more global synthetic role for the right hemisphere. There also appears to be a right parietal dominance for certain emotional aspects of behavior. (5).

4. Semiology: parietal syndrome

The parietal lobe constitutes a veritable crossroads between motor representations and sensory and sensory projections, which explains the richness of the clinical symptomatology. (4).

This syndromic grouping includes sensory disorders, body schema disorders, spatial agnosia, praxis disorders, language disorders, seizures, motor disorders, trophic disorders, memory disorders and personality disorders.

4.1 Sensory disorders:

In the case of parietal lesions, sensory symptoms may be more or less elementary, depending on the location of the lesion.

4.1.1 Lesions of the primary sensory area :

Lesions of the primary sensory area cause superficial hemianesthesia contralateral to the lesion. (2).

- Dejerine and Mouzon syndrome (6) :

It involves contralateral hemianesthesia on the side of the lesion, predominating distally. Stereognosia is affected secondary to anesthesia, while deep sensibility is preserved. The upper limb is most affected. This syndrome is secondary to the interruption of sensory projections following lesions of the post-central gyrus (2).

4.1.2 Lesions of the secondary sensory area :

- Lesions of Brodmann's area 5:

These lesions are responsible for a failure in tactile discrimination. (2):

- *Abarognosia*: the inability to assess the weight of objects
- *Ahylognosia*: The inability to recognize the physical qualities of objects.
- *Amorphognosia*: The inability to recognize the shape of an object by simple manipulation.

➤ Lesions of Brodmann's area 7:

These lesions cause deep sensory damage.

4.1.3 Lesions in tertiary areas:

➤ Astereognosia or secondary tactile agnosia or tactile asymbolia:

This deficit is characterized by the inability to identify an object by simple manipulation, without the aid of sight, in the absence of an elementary sensory deficit or tactile discrimination disorder. In pure astereognosia, evocation of the object's physical qualities is not lost, but cannot be associated with other sensory representations. As a result, object recognition becomes impossible.

➤ Sensitive extinction or *sensitive* inattention:

Appears on bilateral tactile or nociceptive stimulation (2). It is secondary to a lesion of the supra-marginal gyrus.

4.2 Sensory disorders :

➤ Vestibular disorders: with dizziness or a feeling of instability. They may lead to ataxia. These disorders are secondary to lesions of the superior parietal gyrus.

- Taste disorders: characterized by the occurrence of taste hallucinations during lesions of the rolandic operculum. These manifestations are accompanied by paresthesias localized in the lower half of the face and tongue.
- Visual disorders: visual field deficits are linked to damage to the parietal bundle of optic radiations, which reaches the upper lip of the calcarine scissure. This deficit occurs in lesions of the posteroinferior part of the parietal lobe, and is thus responsible for contralateral inferior quadranopsia.

4.3 Body schema disorders:

Body schema refers to the knowledge of the existence of body parts and their spatial relationships.

The supra-marginal area receives visual information from area 7, tactile information from area 5, and limbic input from the posterior cingulate cortex (area 23).

Thus, a lesion in area 40 will lead to body schema disorders.

4.3.1 During lesions of the minor hemisphere :

Signs are unilateral and affect the contralateral hemisphere (the left in right-handed patients). (2,7) :

- Hemi asomatognosia: this is the misrecognition of a hemi-body. Its intensity varies from simple neglect to total unawareness of the hemisphere.

- Anosognosia: manifested by ignorance and refusal to recognize the existence of an obvious disorder, even when it is pointed out to the patient suffering from it. The patient is thus unaware of the paralysis of his or her hemisphere.
- Anosodiaphoria: reflects the patient's indifference to his or her sensory or motor deficit.
- Motor hemi neglect: This is a relatively common disorder, in which the side opposite the brain lesion is ignored. As a result, the patient neglects the use of his or her hemisphere, which can be mobilized if the patient's attention is drawn to it.

4.3.2 In lesions of the dominant hemisphere :

Somatognosia disorders affect both hemispheres(2,7) :

- Autotopoagnosia: This is the inability to locate, and therefore designate, different parts of the body.
- Digital agnosia: This is the inability of a subject to identify his or her fingers or those of the examiner.
- Right-left indistinctness: This is the patient's inability to designate right or left limbs on command.
- Pain asymbolia: Individualized by the perception of elementary painful sensations outside their emotional and affective context: the subject does not perceive their distressing nature, which explains the absence of a normal defense reaction. (8).

4.4 Spatial agnosias or unilateral spatial neglect (NSU):

Concerns recognition of left visual space in right-handed people (2). According to the literature, 85% of patients with a right-hemispheric lesion show signs of NSU.

It can affect reading and writing, as well as more basic activities such as personal care, dressing, getting around and eating. Generally speaking, it reduces patients' autonomy and independence, and is thus a factor with a poor prognosis in functional terms.

NSU is secondary to a lesion of the posterior parietal regions, specifically the supra marginal gyrus of the minor hemisphere (2,9,10).

There are two clinical forms of NSU: corporal neglect and extra-corporal neglect.

4.4.1 Bodily negligence

Neglect of the body can manifest itself as forgetfulness when shaving or applying make-up on the left half of the face (Figure 7**Error! Reference source not found.**), or by stasis of food in the oral cavity during swallowing.

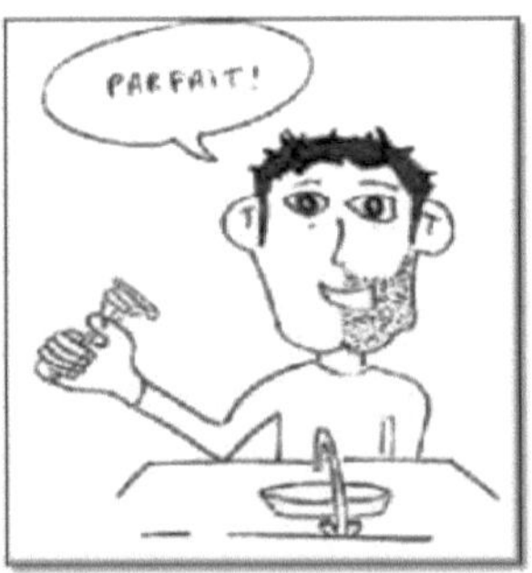

Figure 7Shaving activity in a hemi-careless patient

When the disorder affects the whole hemisphere, it may be revealed by the patient forgetting to use the affected limb, which is usually paralyzed and anesthetized. For example, patients may lie or sit on their upper limb without realizing it. This bodily neglect can be demonstrated by asking the patient to touch different parts of the neglected hemisphere with his or her healthy hand. If there is a deficit, the patient will not be able to reach the target.

4.4.2 Extracorporeal negligence

The deficit is most often seen in the nearby extracorporeal space (Figure 8). The patient thus neglects the various elements in the left hemispace. It is in this part of space that the majority of evaluation tests are performed. The deficit can also affect the distant extracorporeal space.

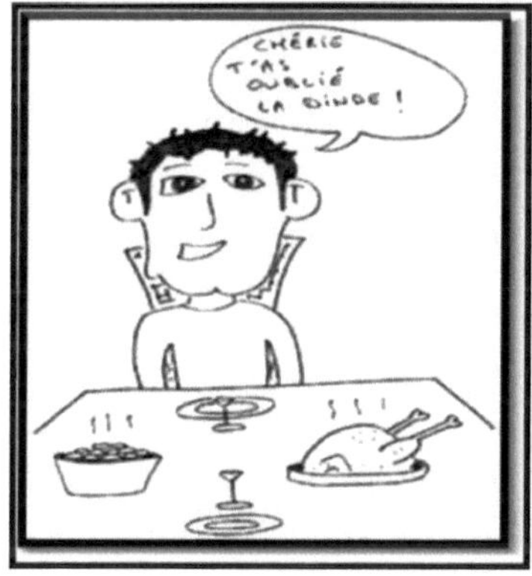

Figure 8 The left extracorporeal negligence

4.4.3 Directional disturbances :

These disturbances are often associated with bodily and extracorporeal negligence. They interfere with movements directed towards the hemispace contralateral to the lesion.

We distinguish :

- Directional hypometry: corresponds to insufficient amplitude of movement towards the side contralateral to the lesion.
- Directional hypokinesia: corresponds to a delay in movement initiation
- Directional bradykinesia: corresponds to slowness in movement execution.

4.5 Visio-spatial disorders:

Problems locating objects in space are most common in bilateral lesions affecting the angular gyrus (11). They have been classified into two categories (2,11):

4.5.1 Absolute localization disorders:

These disorders are characterized by the patient's inability to determine the position in space of objects in relation to his or her own body.

4.5.2 Relative localization disorders:

These disorders are characterized by a poor appreciation of direction and distance. In this sense, the patient has difficulty determining the position and distance between two objects or people in the field of vision.

4.5.3 Clinical implications:

- Of two people in the field of vision, the patient is unable to specify which is closer, or to estimate the distance between them.
- When walking, patients find it difficult to avoid obstacles, and may even run into walls as a result of misjudged distances.
- Patients also show topographical disorientation (they take the wrong direction because they no longer recognize significant landmarks).

4.6 Parietal focal epileptic seizures:

Parietal epileptic seizures are considered rare, accounting for only 5% of surgical series (12). Subjective signs are more specific and common (80% of cases). They are dominated by somato-sensory disturbances, body schema disorders, visual disturbances and vestibular symptoms. (13). The objective semiology of parietal seizures is often misleading, characterized in particular by motor signs linked to the propagation of the discharge.

4.6.1 Subjective semiology :

- Somato-sensory manifestations:

These symptoms occur in 35% to 63% of cases (13). They are essentially represented by paresthesias, more rarely by thermal or painful sensations affecting the contralateral hemisphere, often starting with the hand (14). These manifestations may extend from proximal to proximal. By following the topography of the sensory homonculus, we can localize the lesion clinically, taking into account the onset of the seizure: if paresthesias first appear in the leg, the lesion is localized on the medial side of the parietal lobe. On the other hand, if the seizure starts in the hemiface and hand, the lesion is localized on the outer surface of the contralateral parietal lobe. (2). This focal sensory seizure may radiate to the motor cortex, evolving into a Jacksonian motor seizure. Localized genital sensations suggest that the discharge originates in the paracentral lobule.

- Body schema disorders:

Altered body perception is classically reported during parietal seizures. It is described by around 10% of patients with this type of epileptic seizure. It involves an impression of body shape distortion, elongation or diminution (macro-micro-asomatognosia) of a contralateral limb(15). Unilateral asomatognosia is also possible. These manifestations are secondary to a lesion of the contralateral associative parietal cortex (supra-marginal gyrus) (14).

➢ Visual disorders:

They occur in 10-30% of patients (15). They are essentially visual illusions with changes in the perception of space or objects (15). Out-of-body hallucinations have also been reported during these seizures, and are thought to be related to a lateral parietal origin (16). These phenomena are mainly seen during lesions of the minor hemisphere (13).

➢ Subjective vestibular signs:

These manifestations were reported in 23% of cases (13). They often include sensations of dizziness, falling or tilting. These vestibular symptoms are secondary to lesions of the superior parietal gyrus (15).

4.6.2 Objective manifestations :

The objective semiology classically depends on whether the discharge propagates to the frontal lobe or the temporal lobe (13).

➢ Versive manifestations and ocular signs:

Versive phenomena are among the most frequently encountered manifestations of parietal seizures (41% to 65% of cases). In 70% of cases, they are often limited to a low-tonic orientation of the head and eyes towards the side ipsilateral to the discharge. (13). These phenomena may reflect the involvement of the oculomotor regions of the intraparietal sulcus (17).

- Tonic and clonic manifestations:

Found in 45 to 85% of cases (13). These motor phenomena most often occur in the aftermath of a seizure, but may also be present at the onset of symptomatology (15). In the case of tonic manifestations, the epileptogenic zone is located in the superior parietal gyrus in 61% of cases. In fact, this convolution projects extensively into the pre-motor cortex (area 6 and supplementary motor area) (14).

- Gestural or oral automatisms:

17% of patients with parietal seizures have gestural or oral automatisms, and 4% have complex automatisms (14). In 79% of these patients, the epileptogenic zone is located in the inferior parietal gyrus. Indeed, ECs originating in this area will most often diffuse to the temporo-limbic structures (14).

4.7 Praxis disorders:

Apraxia is a deficit characterized by the inability to perform certain movements voluntarily, despite the preservation of motility, sensitivity, coordination and the ability to understand language(18). It is mainly characterized by automatic-voluntary dissociation, since the same gestures can be performed automatically. The disorder does not affect a unitary movement, but a coordinated action based on a result or intention.

The deficit therefore lies at the psychophysiological level of initiation and execution of the voluntary motor actor. (19).

The praxis disorders observed are of different types:

4.7.1 *Ideomotor apraxia :*

Ideomotor apraxia refers to the inability to perform gestures on command that do not require the use of an object. The gestures concerned are either intransitive (without the use of an object) or transitive (mimicking the use of an object).
In this type of apraxia, the subject is incapable of arranging, one after the other, the different times of movement to perform the act in question, while retaining the concept of the act to be performed (2,18). Gestures are thus clumsy, approximate or erroneous. One action may be substituted for another, or the patient may verbalize the action he or she cannot perform, or use body parts as objects (brushing teeth with fingers).

- Bilateral ideomotor apraxia: associated with lesions of the inferior parietal gyrus, and especially the left supra-marginal gyrus in right-handed patients (2,20).
- Unilateral ideomotor apraxia: observed in lesions of the inferior parietal gyrus of the minor hemisphere and affecting the contralateral hemisphere (2,20).

4.7.2 *Ideatory apraxia*

In ideatory apraxia, the patient has lost the concept of the nature of the act to be performed. It affects the ability to manipulate objects (18). This type of apraxia affects complex acts, as the subject can neither program nor coordinate the elementary gestures that constitute it, whereas the latter are correctly executed if taken in isolation (18). This disorder is linked to lesions of the left temporo-parieto-occipital carrefour (20).

Example: It is very difficult for a person suffering from ideatory apraxia to insert a key into a lock, peel a piece of fruit, light a candle... Gestures are clumsy and confused.

4.7.3 Constructive apraxia:

This apraxia consists of difficulty in putting together one-dimensional units to form two- or multi-dimensional figures. It is sought either by drawing, or with sticks or matches (21). The subject is unable to assemble straight lines to form a square, triangle or cube.

This type of apraxia is associated with a right, left or bilateral posterior parietal lesion. (2).

- Right-sided lesions:

The deficit is visuo-spatial. Programming of the whole constructive activity is possible, but there are difficulties in recognizing the component parts of the whole, with difficulties in comparing the model with the actual performance. As a result, the lines are misdirected, sometimes with unnecessary details added. (22).

- Left lesions:

The basic deficit is that resulting from the implementation of the business plan. (23). The construction task is carried out step by step, and drawing is simplified (24).

4.7.4 *Apraxia of dressing :*

This disorder consists of difficulty in orienting clothing in relation to the body: the patient handles clothing incoherently, making mistakes and trying things out unsuccessfully. This apraxia is observed in lesions of the minor hemisphere.

4.8 Language disorders :

Since 1914, Dejerine has proposed the left angular gyrus as "a center of visual word images" (Figure 9) (6). Since then, the left parietal lobe has been implicated in the genesis of language disorders. Lesions of the left angular gyrus, left supra-marginal gyrus or subcortical white matter may be the cause.

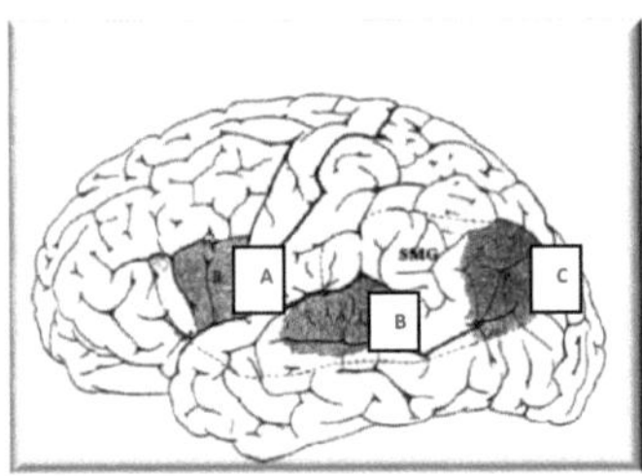

Figure 9The language centers of the left hemisphere according to Dejerine 1914: A: Broca's area; B: Wernicke's area; C: angular gyrus.

4.8.1 *Lesions of the left angular gyrus:*

Are responsible for agraphia with verbal blindness (alexia) (6) :

- Agraphia: is characterized by spelling errors, deformations and word substitutions (paragraphing). It affects spontaneous, copied and dictated writing.
- Alexia: rarely isolated in parietal syndromes; associated with agraphia in lesions of the left curved fold, or occurring as part of Wernicke's aphasia.

4.8.2 Lesions of the left supra marginal gyrus

These lesions are responsible for transcortical sensory aphasia and conduction aphasia. (2) :

- Transcortical sensory aphasia: characterized by fluent spontaneous language, with paraphasia and sometimes jargon, a comprehension deficit and normal repetition.
- Conduction aphasia: is secondary to interruption of the arcuate bundle that connects Broca's and Wernicke's areas (Figure 10). This aphasia occurs in lesions involving the anterior parietal cortex or the left supra-marginal gyrus. It affects sentence programming. Oral and written language comprehension is normal. The disorder mainly manifests itself in reading aloud, writing under dictation and repeating sentences, with, in these cases, the occurrence of paraphasia and word telescoping. It is therefore a language disorder that appears when moving from one type of information to a different type of production.

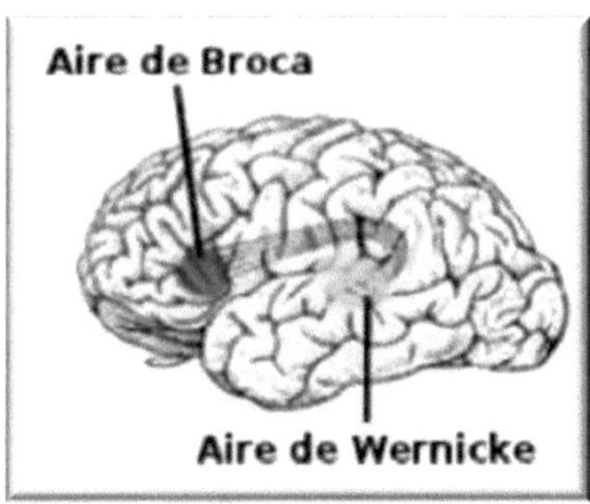

Figure 10The arcuate bundle pathway linking Broca's and Wernicke's areas

4.8.3 Lesions of the left angular gyrus and supra-marginal gyrus:

➢ Wernicke's aphasia :

Linked to a lesion of Wernicke's area, which includes the supra-marginal gyrus and the curved fold. It is characterized by severe impairment of comprehension, with verbal expression using inappropriate words, giving the impression that the patient is using his own jargon. One of the most important features of Wernicke's aphasia is exaggerated fluency. Associated with this are articulation disorders, the production of a large number of paraphrases, generally meaningless language and significant comprehension disorders.

4.8.4 Lesions of the temporao-parietal junction :

➢ Amnesic aphasia or lack of *words* (25)Amnesic aphasia: occurs in naming and spontaneous speech. It affects word selection, while articulation and syntax are normal, and oral and written comprehension are good. The patient replaces the unrecognized word with a periphrase (instead of saying "pencil", he says "it's for writing").

4.9 Motor disorders :

4.9.1 Motor deficiency :

Found only in fronto-parietal lesions involving the ascending frontal convolution.

4.9.2 Motor hemi-aspontaneities:

Secondary to motor neglect. In this disorder, there is a tendency towards catatonic postures of the affected limb, and a certain degree of hypotonia rather than spasticity.

4.9.3 Parietal ataxia

It has been shown that, in addition to lesions of the cerebellum and brainstem, lesions of the parietal lobe can be responsible for ataxia (26,27).

This ataxia is secondary to damage to Brodmann's area 5. This area receives and transmits the majority of cerebellar projections via the ventrolateral nucleus of the thalamus and the pontine nuclei (Figure 11) (26-28).

The static component of parietal ataxia has been described as "unstable ataxic hand" (21).

The kinetic component can be demonstrated in the finger-on-finger test with eyes closed. In this test, the "seeking" finger (on the diseased side) is difficult to reach. Less often, the "seeking" finger (on the diseased side) hesitates before reaching the "seeking" finger (on the healthy side). This situation is secondary to a poor appreciation of the movement's coordinates in space (21).

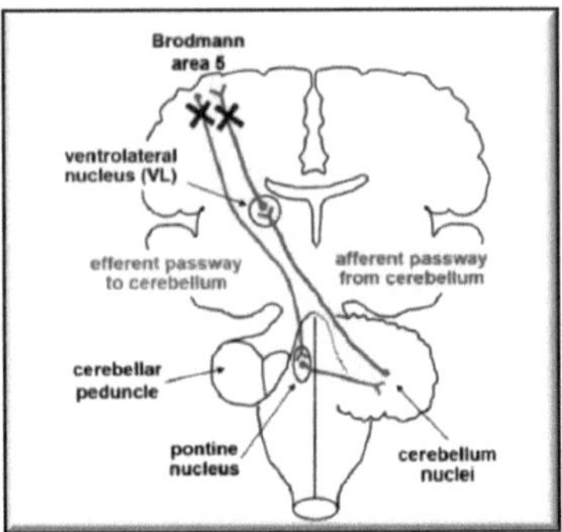

Figure 11Theoretical model of parietal ataxia: Brodmann's area 5 is the main area that sends projections to the cerebellum via the pontine nucleus and receives afferents from the cerebellum via the ventro-lateral nucleus of the thalamus.

4.9.4 *Ataxic hemiparesis*

This is a hemiparesis accompanied by a cerebellar-like ataxia on the side contralateral to the lesion. This syndrome is secondary to lesions of the parietal subcortical white matter, following damage to corticospinal and parietopontine fibers at various levels of the central nervous system. (29).

4.10 Trophic disorders:

This is an amyotrophy affecting the contralateral upper limb, either at the root or distal end. Electromyographic examination is normal. Amyotrophy is always accompanied by major hypotonia (2,30). This type of amyotrophy occurs mainly in cases of post-central gyrus tumours (2,31).

4.11 Memory disorders:

The parietal lobe plays an important role in memory processes. Indeed, several studies have shown that lesions of the parietal lobe, and particularly of the left angular gyrus, determine episodic memory disorders, affecting both the encoding and retrieval processes (32). Other studies have incriminated lesions of the posterior parietal lobe in working memory deficits (33).

4.12 Personality disorders:

Parietal lesions can profoundly alter the patient's personality. Indeed, the inferior parietal gyrus and the temporo-parietal junction of the two hemispheres can be the source of a number of symptoms such as: auditory and visual hallucinations, bizarre behavior, thought disorders with delusions of persecution, jealousy or reference, social isolation or aggressiveness (33). Thus, schizophrenia, depression, bipolar disorders and psychomotor instability may be the result of inferior parietal lesions (33). Acute confusional states have also been reported in infarcts of the posterior territory of the right middle cerebral artery .

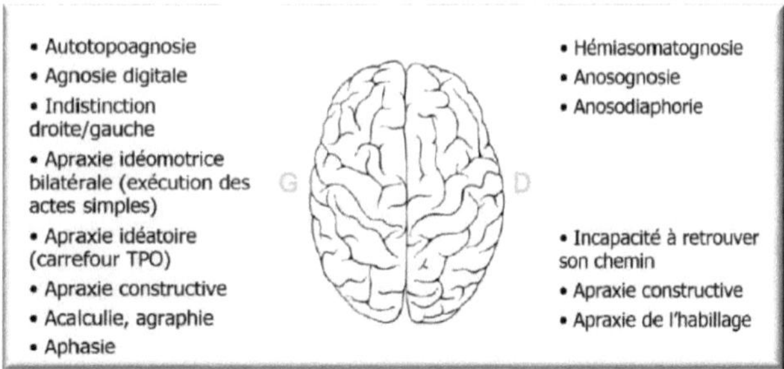

Figure 12Hemispheric differences

4.13 Clinical forms

Clinical symptomatology depends on the location of the lesion in the parietal lobe, and whether neighbouring structures are affected. A number of clinical syndromes have been identified:

4.13.1 Gerstmann syndrome (2,34) :

This syndrome is linked to a lesion of the angular gyrus of the dominant hemisphere. It includes digital agnosia, right-left indistinction, acalculia and pure agraphia, frequently with constructive apraxia.

4.13.2 Right parieto-occipital syndrome in right-handed people:

It is characterized by spatial disorganization, and includes constructive apraxia, dressing apraxia, unilateral left-sided spatial agnosia, and disorders of topographical memory and orientation.

4.13.3 Balint syndrome (35-37) :

This is a characteristic triad of symptoms, each of which can occur in isolation: psychic paralysis of the gaze, optic ataxia and simultagnosia.

- Psychic gaze paralysis: is defined by the patient's inability to direct his gaze towards a target in his visual field. Pursuit movements are abolished and disturbed, while automatic-reflex eye movements are normal. This disorder is secondary to a lesion of the inferior parietal gyrus, since the control and triggering of visually guided saccades is located in the upper part of area 39.

- Optic ataxia: defined as the inability to accurately perform a manual input under visual guidance in a hemi visual field in the absence of sensory-motor, cerebellar, extrapyramidal deficits or hemianopia.
- Simultagnosia: the patient is unable to see two objects at the same time. If he sees the object placed in the fovea, he recognizes it correctly, but is unable to detect a second target presented simultaneously just a few centimetres from the first.

4.13.4 Anton Babinski syndrome:

This is a major form of hemi asomatognosia associated with anosognosia and hemiplegia. This syndrome is often associated with hemianesthesia. Patients may exhibit delusional behavior in relation to the left hemisphere, going so far as to tap or cut the paralyzed side that encumbers them.

5. Clinical examination :

5.1 Sensitivity test :

5.1.1 Search for sensitive extinction :

During isolated stimulation (tactile or puncture) of the right or left side of the body, the patient (eyes closed) is aware of the intensity and location of the stimulus. On the other hand, when such stimulation is applied simultaneously to both sides of the body, the same patient recognizes only the stimulation applied to the healthy hemisphere.

5.1.2 Searching for a tactile discrimination disorder: the Weber circle :

We place the two points of a compass on a part of the patient's body. This will determine the minimum space where the patient feels two distinct points. In parietal syndrome, the distance required for discrimination between these two points is markedly increased in the hemisphere contralateral to the lesion.

5.2 The search for unilateral spatial agnosia :

5.2.1 Patient inspection :

NSU may be evident on inspection of the patient. In the usual form, the patient presents a permanent head and gaze deviation to the right. He ignores stimuli coming from the side contralateral to the brain lesion. When walking, the right leg is always brought forward, while the other is left behind.

5.2.2 NSU tests and assessment tools

Several diagnostic tests have been proposed for assessing spatial neglect:

- Copying drawings :

Patients with a lesion of the right supra-marginal gyrus show a spatial neglect that is evident in spontaneous or copied drawing. They omit or distort elements located on the left. Some patients present an object-centered NSU phenomenon, in which all elements are present but the left part of an item may be missing (Figure 13).

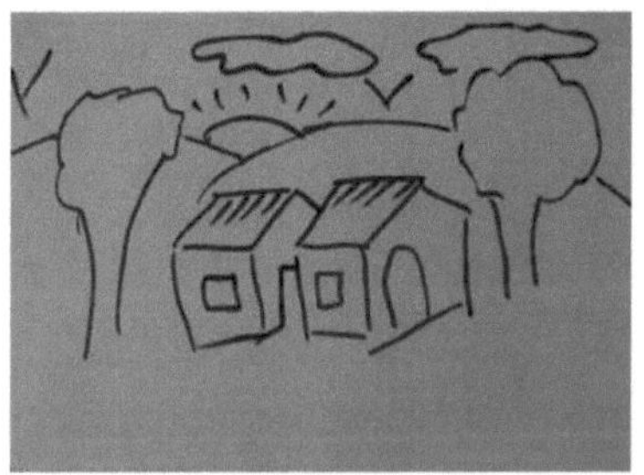

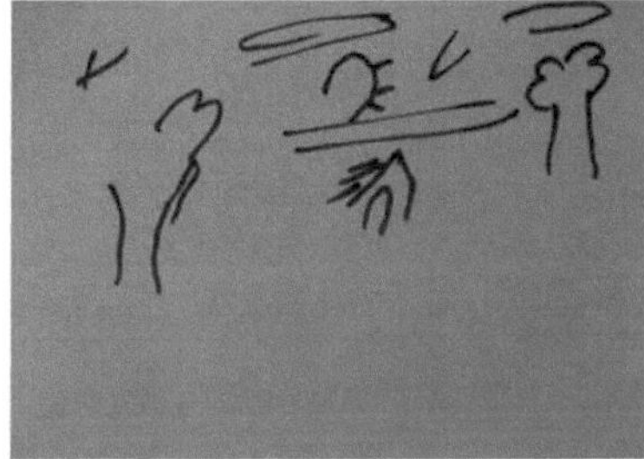

Figure 13The drawing copy test in a hemi-neglect patient

- <u>Writing and reading</u>

The hemi-neglecting patient writes on the right half of the sheet with less legible handwriting (Figure 14).

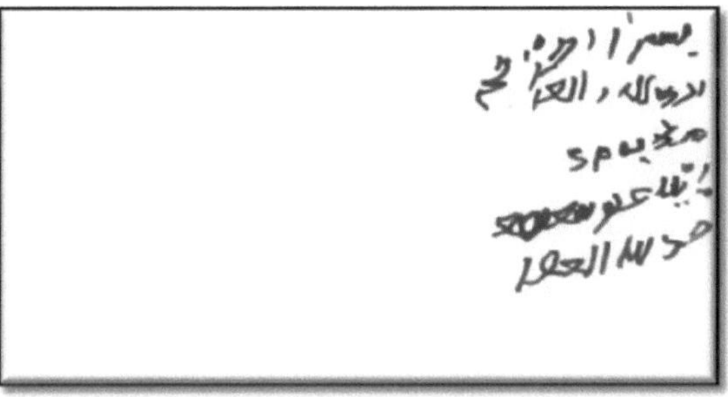

Figure 14Handwriting test in a hemi-neglect patient

When reading a book or newspaper, the patient focuses on the right-hand side and omits the left-hand side.

- <u>The barrage test :</u>

Patients are asked to tick or circle lines, letters and shapes. They usually start exploring on the right-hand side and omit elements on the left.

- <u>The bell test</u>

This is the most widely used test for evaluating NSU.

In the bells test, the patient is asked to use a pen to circle the 35 bells contained on an A4 sheet of paper among 280 other figurines. All the figures are in black. The sheet is placed in front of the patient. The bells are distributed randomly among all the figurines. They are divided into 7 columns. Each column contains 5 bells and 40 other figures.

The total number of bells circled will be noted, as well as the time it took the patient to perform it.

The maximum score is 35. Missing 6 or more bells indicates the presence of NSU. The spatial distribution of missed bells enables the examiner to assess the severity and laterality of visual neglect (Figure 15). The sequence in which the patient completed this task can be represented by connecting the circled bells with lines, following the order in which the patient performed the task.

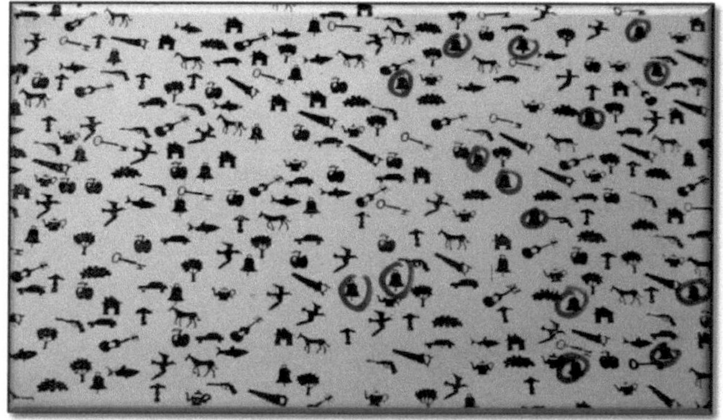

Figure 15 The bell test showing the presence of left-sided spatial neglect

- The line bisection test:

This is a frequently requested test for the detection of NSU. When patients are asked to indicate the midpoint of horizontal lines of different lengths, they neglect the lines to the left and deviate the subjective midpoint of each line to the right (Figure 16).

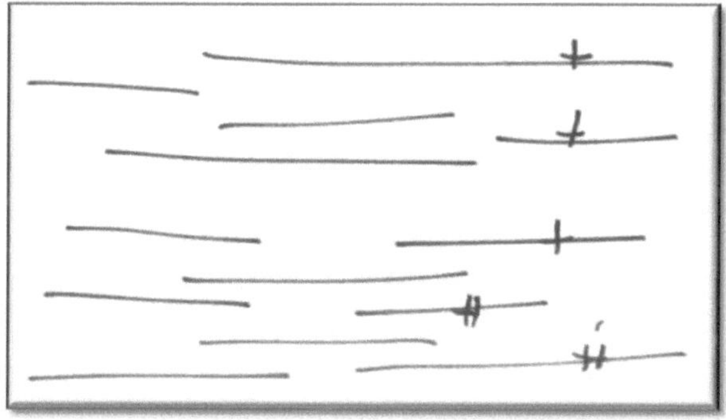

Figure 16 The line bisection test in a hemi-neglect patient

- Entangled figures

Patients have to name the different objects that are in parts superimposed: 2 on the left, one in the middle and 2 on the right. Some patients will omit the items on the left.

Sometimes, even without omission, there is a clear tendency for patients to name the items on the right first (Figure 17).

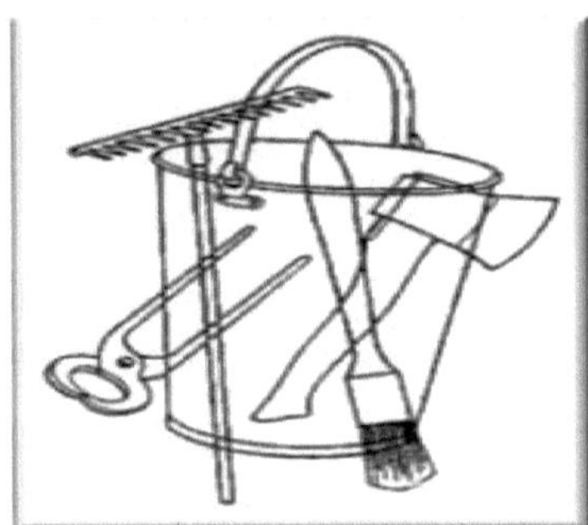

Figure 17 : Example of interlocking figures

- ➢ The clock test:

The clock test is a simple, rapid test for detecting spatial neglect. The patient is asked to correctly place the digits inside the clock face, and the spatial distribution of these digits (right and left) is examined. To do this, we draw a circle 10 cm in diameter, place it in front of the patient and ask him/her to write the hour digits (from 1 to 12) inside this clock.

Assessment:

- ✓ Overall score: The evaluation is semi-quantitative with a 3-level scale:
    - 0: clock face correctly completed
    - 1: incomplete dial on left
    - 2: no dial digits on the left

- ✓ Completion time (in seconds)
- ✓ Interpretation: the test is considered pathological if the overall score > 0 or the time > 70 seconds (Figure 18).

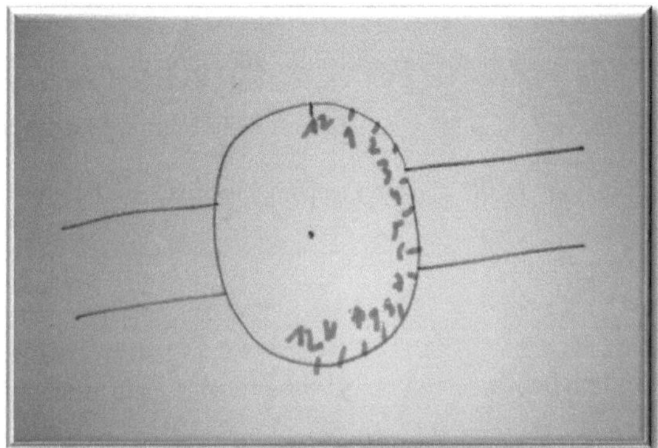

Figure 18Clock test performed by a patient with left-sided spatial neglect

5.3 The search for ideomotor apraxia:

The brief battery for assessing gestural praxis, developed by Florence Mahieux in 2008 (38) (appendix), is a protocol designed to assess gestural praxias of the upper limbs. It tests symbolic gestures (e.g. military salute), abstract gestures (e.g. putting the palm of the right hand on the right cheek), and action mimes (e.g. driving a nail with a hammer). For each of these gesture categories, the instructions and scoring system are different.

- ✓ For symbolic gestures, the patient is asked: "Show me how you do it...". The participant's productions are scored out of zero or one point. A point is awarded if the gesture is generally recognizable. The maximum score is 5. For this domain, a threshold score of 4/5 has been proposed.

- ✓ For action mime gestures, the patient is asked: "Imagine you're holding a... in your hand, show me the gesture you make to...". Three scores can be given: zero, one or two. Two points correspond to correct execution of the gesture, one point corresponds to persistent assimilation of the body to the object on one side, and zero points correspond to a bad gesture or bimanual assimilation of the body to the object. Assimilation of the body to the object" means using a part of the body to represent the object, e.g. using the finger as a match rather than pretending to hold a match. The maximum mark is 10. It has been suggested that performance should be considered "out of the ordinary" when the subject achieves a score of less than 8/10.
- ✓ Finally, participants are asked to perform the abstract gestures in imitation. The examiner explains, "I'm going to ask you to make exactly the same gesture as me, with the same hand as me. In the event of a mirror-image error, you can ask "Are you sure? Is this the same hand as mine? Participants' gestures are scored as zero or one point. The point is awarded if the participant ends up doing it correctly, even after the instruction has been recalled or after the examiner has provided support in the case of mirrored production. The maximum mark is 8. It has been suggested that performance be considered "abnormal" for a score below 7/8 for patients under 65 and 6/8 for patients over 65.

Conclusion

Lésion		Droit	Gauche
Gyrus pariétal ascendant		▪ Hémianesthésie controlatérale à la lésion ▪ Crises épileptiques sensitives ▪ Troubles trophiques du membre supérieur controlatéral à la lésion	
Gyrus pariétal supérieur	AB 5	▪ Troubles de la discrimination tactile ▪ Ataxie pariétale ▪ Crises épileptique (troubles vestibulaires)	
	AB 7	▪ Troubles de la proprioception	
Gyrus pariétal inférieur	AB 39	▪ Troubles visio-spatiaux	▪ Troubles visio-spatiaux ▪ Agraphie ▪ Alexie ▪ Troubles de la mémoire épisodique ▪ Syndrome de Gerstmann ▪ Apraxie idéatoire
	AB 40	▪ Hémi asomatognosie ▪ Anosognosie ▪ Anosodiaphorie ▪ Hémi négligence motrice ▪ Négligence spatiale unilatérale ▪ Extinction sensitive ▪ Apraxie d'habillage ▪ Apraxie constructive	▪ Auto-topoagnosie ▪ Agnosie digitale ▪ Indistinction droite-gauche ▪ Asymbolie à la douleur ▪ Aphasie transcorticale sensorielle ▪ Aphasie de conduction ▪ Extinction sensitive ▪ Apraxie idéo-motrice ▪ Apraxie constructive

References

1. Caspers S, Zilles K. Microarchitecture and connectivity of the parietal lobe. Handb Clin Neurol. 2018;151:53-72.

2. Berlucchi G, Vallar G. The history of the neurophysiology and neurology of the parietal lobe. Handb Clin Neurol. 2018;151:3–30.

3. Vogt C, Vogt O. Allgemeinere Ergebnisse Unserer Hirnforschung. J Psychol Neurol. 1919;25: 279-461.

4. Kim Y-H, Kim JS, Lee SK, Chung CK. Neurologic Outcome After Resection of Parietal Lobe Including Primary Somatosensory Cortex: Implications of Additional Resection of Posterior Parietal Cortex. World Neurosurg. 2017;106:884–90.

5. Lehman Blake M. Clinical relevance of discourse characteristics after right hemisphere brain damage. Am J Speech Lang Pathol. 2006;15(3):255–67.

6. Dejerine J (1914). S_emiologie des affections du syste`me nerveux. Masson, Paris.

7. Vallar G, Maravita A (2009). Personal and extra-personal spatial perception. In: GG Berntson, JT Cacioppo (Eds.), Handbook of neuroscience for the behavioral sciences. John Wiley, New York, pp. 322-336. In.

8. Schilder P (1935). The image and appearance of the human body. International Universities Press, New York.

9. Benton AL, Sivan AB (1992). Neurological examination: double simultaneous stimulation. In: B Smith, G Edelman (Eds.), Neuroscience year: supplement 2 to the encyclopedia of neuroscience. Springer Science and Business Media, New York, pp. 115-116.

10. Paterson A, Zangwill OL (1944). Disorders of visual space perception associated with lesions of the right cerebral hemisphere. Brain 67: 331-335.

11. Holmes G, Horrax G (1919). Disturbances of spatial orientation and visual attention with loss of stereoscopic vision. Arch Neurol Psychiatry 1: 385-407.

12. Kim DW, Lee SK, Yun C-H, Kim K-K, Lee DS, Chung C-K, et al. Parietal lobe epilepsy: the semiology, yield of diagnostic workup, and surgical outcome. Epilepsia. 2004;45(6):641–9.

13. Bartolomei F. Les épilepsies pariétales: cadres nosologiques et sémiologie. Prat Neurol - FMC. 2015;6(2):97–102.

14. Salanova V. Parietal lobe epilepsy. Handb Clin Neurol. 2018;151:413–25.

15. Bartolomei F, Gavaret M, Hewett R, Valton L, Aubert S, Régis J, et al. Neural networks underlying parietal lobe seizures: a quantified study from intracerebral recordings. Epilepsy Res. 2011;93(2-3):164–76.

16. Blanke O, Landis T, Spinelli L, Seeck M. Out-of-body experience and autoscopy of neurological origin. Brain J Neurol. 2004;127(Pt 2):243–58.

17. Grefkes C, Fink GR. The functional organization of the intraparietal sulcus in humans and monkeys. J Anat. 2005;207(1):3–17.

18. Buxbaum LJ, Randerath J. Limb apraxia and the left parietal lobe. Handb Clin Neurol. 2018;151:349–63.

19. Peigneux P, Van der Linden M, Garraux G, Laureys S, Degueldre C, Aerts J, et al. Imaging a cognitive model of apraxia: the neural substrate of gesture-specific cognitive processes. Hum Brain Mapp. 2004;21(3):119–42.

20. Liepmann H (1920). Apraxia. Ergebnisse der gesamten Medizin 1: 516-543.

21. Critchley M. The parietal lobes. Oxford, England: Williams and Wilkins; 1953. vii, 480 (The parietal lobes).

22. Benton AL. Visuoconstructive disability in patients with cerebral disease: Its relationship to side of lesion and aphasic disorder. Doc Ophthalmol. 1973;34(1):67-76.

23. HECAEN H, ALBERT ML. Human neuropsychology. John Wiley and Sons. New York. 1978; pp 94-138, 176-225, 277-297.

24. BOTEZ MI, BOTEZ T, OLIVIER M. Parietal lobe syndromes. In: Fredericks JAM ed. Handbook of clinical neurology, vol 45. Elsevier Science Publishers. Amsterdam. 1985 ; pp 63-85.

25. Luria AR, Sokolov EN, Klimkowski M (). Towards a neurodynamic analysis of memory disturbances with lesions of the left temporal lobe. Neuropsychologia. 1967;5: 1-11.

26. Futamura A, Kawamura M. Parietal Ataxia: 13 Cases Plus a Review of Relevant Literature. Showa Univ J Med Sci. 2014;26(4):263–9.

27. Morihara R, Yamashita T, Deguchi K, Kurata T, Nomura E, Sato K, et al. Familial and sporadic chronic progressive degenerative parietal ataxia. J Neurol Sci. 2018;387:70–4.

28. Hyvärinen J. Posterior parietal lobe of the primate brain. Physiol Rev. 1982;62(3):1060–129.

29. SAITOH H, SHINOHARA Y, YOSHII F, YAZAKI K Ataxic hemisparesis due to small semioval center infarction. Tokai J Exp Clin Med 1991; 16: 157-161.

30. Botez MI. Some Clinical Findings Concerning Muscular Atrophy of Central Origin. Eur Neurol. 1971;5(1):25–33.

31. Silverstein A (1955). Diagnostic localizing value of muscle atrophy in parietal lobe lesions. Neurology 5: 30.

32. Rugg MD, King DR. Ventral lateral parietal cortex and episodic memory retrieval. Cortex J Devoted Study Nerv Syst Behav (2017).

33. Teixeira S, Machado S, Velasques B, Sanfim A, Minc D, Peressutti C, et al. Integrative parietal cortex processes: neurological and psychiatric aspects. J Neurol Sci. 2014;338(1-2):12–22.

34. Gerstmann J (1942). Problem of imperception of disease and of impaired body territories with organic lesions. Arch Neurol Psychiatry 48: 890-913.

35. Balint R (1909). Seelenleahmung des "Schauens," optische Ataxie, reaumliche Steorung der Aufmerksamkeit. Monatschrift feur Psychiatrie und Neurologie 25: 51-81.

36. Chechlacz M. Bilateral parietal dysfunctions and disconnections in simultanagnosia and Bálint syndrome. Handb Clin Neurol. 2018;151:249–67.

37. Hausser CO, Robert F, Giard N. Balint's syndrome. Can J Neurol Sci J Can Sci Neurol. 1980;7(2):157–61.

38. Mahieux-Laurent F, Fabre C, Galbrun E, Dubrulle A, Moroni C, Groupe de réflexion sur les praxies du CMRR Ile-de-France Sud. [Validation of a brief screening scale evaluating praxic abilities for use in memory clinics. Evaluation in 419 controls, 127 mild cognitive impairment and 320 demented patients]. Rev Neurol (Paris). Jul 2009;165(6–7):560–7.

Appendix

Annexe A. Batterie brève d'évaluation des praxies gestuelles.

Praxies gestuelles symboliques

CONSIGNE :

Dire: « *Montrez-moi comment vous faites avec la main (le doigt) pour…* »

Faire un salut militaire (français) :	0/1
Demander le silence : « Chut ! » : mauvais/bon	0/1
Montrer que ça sent mauvais (ça pue) : mauvais/bon	0/1
Dire que quelqu'un est fou : mauvais/bon	0/1
Envoyer un baiser : mauvais/bon	0/1

NOTATION :

Le geste est considéré comme bon, s'il est globalement reconnaissable par un observateur extérieur ; score total : /5

Praxies gestuelles mimes d'action

CONSIGNE :

Dire: « *Imaginez que vous tenez dans la main un…, montrez-moi le geste que vous faites pour…* » ; on peut préciser : « *Voilà un* (faire semblant de donner l'objet), *montrez-moi le geste que vous faites pour …* » en cas d'assimilation du corps à l'objet, on peut rappeler la consigne initiale ou dire : « *Montrez-moi comment vous tenez le… ?* »

Normal = 2 ; assimilation persistante du corps à l'objet d'un côté = 1 ; mauvais geste ou assimilation du corps à l'objet bimanuelle = 0

Planter un clou avec un marteau:	0/1/2
Déchirer en deux une feuille de papier :	0/1/2
Allumer une allumette :	0/1/2
Vous peigner les cheveux avec un peigne :	0/1/2
Boire un verre :	0/1/2

NOTATION :

Le geste est considéré comme bon, s'il est globalement reconnaissable par un observateur extérieur, les mains laissant la place pour l'objet imaginaire (score unitaire de 2). En cas d'assimilation du corps à l'objet pour une seule main ou de geste imparfait mais reconnaissable, score de 1, si le geste n'est pas reconnaissable ou qu'il y a assimilation bimanuelle, score unitaire de 0 ; score total : /10

Gestes abstraits

CONSIGNE :

Dire: « *Je vais vous demander de faire exactement le même geste que moi, avec la même main que moi, c'est-à-dire avec votre main droite si je le fais de la main droite et avec votre main gauche, si je le fais de la main gauche* ».

Le geste doit être maintenu jusqu'à ce que le patient l'ait reproduit ou qu'il soit évident qu'il ne peut y arriver. En cas d'erreur « en miroir » demander « *Êtes-vous bien sûr ? Est-ce la même main que moi ?* »

Les mains doivent revenir sur la table entre chaque geste. Les gestes sont montrés sur la Fig. 1.

On peut éventuellement (papillon, double anneau), montrer la dynamique du geste.

Paume de la main droite sur la joue droite	0/1
Dos de la main droite sur la joue controlatérale gauche:	0/1
Paume de la main gauche sur la joue gauche	0/1
Dos de la main gauche sur la joue controlatérale gauche :	0/1
Mains sur la table, droite à plat, gauche faisant les cornes des doigts II–V :	0/1
Papillon :	0/1
Losange II–III (mains inversées, perpendiculaire à la table : en l'air et pas à plat) :	0/1
Double anneau :	0/1

NOTATION :

Le geste est bon si le patient finit par le faire correctement, même après rappel de la consigne.

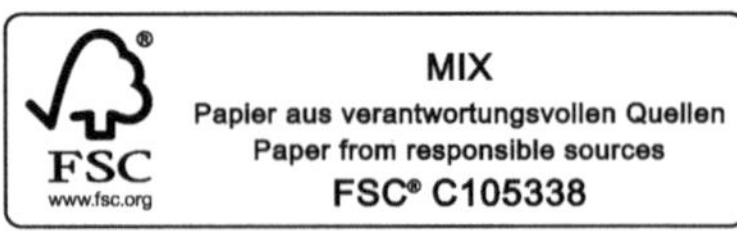

Printed by Books on Demand GmbH, Norderstedt / Germany